How To Start Your Personal Training Business

Step by Step Business Plan and Forms

Joe Dynasty

Author Online!
For updates visit Joe Dynasty page at

www.personaltrainerjob.com

How To Start Your Personal Training Business
by **Joe Dynasty**

ISBN 978-0-9866004-3-2

Printed in the United States of America

Copyright © 2010 Psylon Press

Contents

Chapter 1

Right Time, Right Place

If you thought that personal training was only for the rich and the famous, think again! The huge demand for personal trainers today is brought on by more and more regular Americans seeking personal trainer to help them with their fitness routines.

Weighed down by their sedentary lifestyles, Americans of all ages are all looking to reduce the ill effects of hours spent in front of the computer or televisions. Parents want to be healthy role models for their children. Senior citizens want to cut healthcare costs through exercise and diet. And employers would like to increase employee productivity through fitness.

Clearly, this is no fitness craze. And with statistics indicating that personal training is the fastest- growing segment of the fitness industry, savvy entrepreneur like you will know that getting into an expanding career field gives you the advantage of rising faster in the industry.

So, if you are dedicated to the pursuit of a healthy and fit society, now is the time to make your move.

What Do Personal Trainers Do?

Personal trainers are exercise professionals. They work one-on-one with their clients (very rarely also with small groups or couples) to:

- Identify fitness needs of the client

- Establish short-term and long-term goals

- Develop individualized fitness programs

- Teach effective exercise techniques

- Monitor, record and evaluate progress

- Revise the exercise routine as required

- Support and motivate their client to stick to the program and reach their goals

How Do I Know This Is the Right Fit For Me?

• Are you passionate about health and fitness?

• Do you update yourself on the latest trends in health, nutrition and exercise?

• Do you enjoy training others, and guiding them to reach their fitness goals?

• Do you follow a fitness regimen yourself?

• Are you a self-starter?

• Do you think you have patience and empathy?

•Are you friendly, enthusiastic and have great communication skills?

•Are you confident?

•Do you like the idea of being in control of your time?

•Do you agree that rather than selling a service, you are helping people?

•Do you have strong management, administrative and marketing skills?

If you have answered these questions in the affirmative, congratulations! You are bang on target about starting off as a personal trainer.

Chapter 2

Be Your Own Boss

We all know that running a successful business isn't easy; otherwise all exercise professionals would be personal trainers. So why would you risk your little paycheck at the end of the month?

While some of you might want to strike out on your own to escape a badly paid Gym job, others might go solo in search of a flexible career that allows them to do something they enjoy, and some others might be driven by a to be their own boss.

Whatever your motivation, here are the top reasons that will tell you that you are on the right track.

Do What You're Interested In

Do you dream of training elite athletes instead of the elderly population that forms the bulk of the clientele at the gym where you work? If you would rather be doing something else, go solo! As an entrepreneur you can choose what kind of customer profile you are looking for. So, providing that you've done your research properly and there is a gap in the market, you can turn your dream into a profitable enterprise.

Be Your Own Boss

Do you feel you are stuck in a job you loath with a manager who is giving you a hard time? In business, the only person you have to answer to is yourself. Being your own boss gives you the freedom to do things your way and implement your own plans.

Huge Income Potential

When you work in a health club, you probably get paid by the hour. And your employer controls how many hours/sessions you work. But, in your personal training business, you are the boss. You get to decide how many sessions you will conduct each day, and how much you will charge your clients. Although the startup process can be tough, if you run your business well, the rewards can be huge (and you will get most of the profits yourself).

Flexibility

Every one of us, at some point, has dreamed of the freedom to work our own hours. Now you can schedule your training sessions around your kid's football match, and no-one would object!

Variety Is the Spice of Life

Do you enjoy multi-tasking? Then you are going to enjoy the quicksilver role change that your business will demand from you. You will be dealing with spreadsheets one minute, customers the next, just as equipment vendors come calling to do up your swanky new studio. There is no scope of monotony setting in your busy life now.

Recognition

Nothing boosts your morale as getting the credit for your efforts. And as the good word spreads, so does your client base!

Sense of Accomplishment

Finally, nothing excites an enterprising soul more than an expanding bottom-line! New clients, growing business, and health returns for your hard work – that's the motivation for a true entrepreneur.

Turn Your Big Dream Into Reality

If you are being put down by skeptic souls who feel that starting up a small firm won't lead to anything big, share with them the story of Richard Branson. Don't let your dream die because someone somewhere sees it as mere fantasy. Only you can turn your dream into reality. Just make sure that you are well-equipped to manage your business well, and then there's no stopping you.

Chapter 3

License to Train

Now that you have made your decision, the first milestone in your road map should be to get certified. Based on your interests, and the market needs of the area you are going to operate in, you will probably have identified an area of specialization, such as working with pre-natal women or helping people to lose weight. Now, you must now focus on how to get the training and qualifications you need.

Why Should I Get Certified?

You wouldn't allow an unqualified dentist to work on your teeth, or employ an uncertified mechanic to fix your car. So why would you want an uncertified person to work on your fitness routine? Obviously, certification is crucial.

In an increasingly complex and highly-specialized market, credentials are everything. You know that you've got the skills to do the job, but how do you convince potential customers and employers? As a certified fitness professional, you are on par with an industry standard. Your certification assures the client that you possess a certain level of knowledge and that they can rely on you to train them.

Proper qualifications ensure that you obtain the relevant expertise as a professional trainer, and that you are able to offer the best possible exercise solutions to your clients. And equally importantly, these credentials testify that you have the right training to help others train. When a prospective client sees the letters 'CPT' after your name, they see you as the right choice to put their fitness schedules on track.

How Do I Get Certified?

When you look for certification, look for organization with accreditation from the National Commission for Certifying Agencies (NCCA). This is the gold standard achievement in the fitness and allied health professions in US.

If you are not living in US, you can search for 'personal trainer certification country name' in Google or other search engine.

The challenge for you is to find the right certification. Imagine spending hundreds of dollars and endless hours on a certification that lets you work with a specific population when you would rather be working with general, healthy population.

Remember, there are hundreds of certifications that you could choose from, but only a dozen or so are NCCA accredited. To choose the right certification for your personal trainer endeavor,

• Find out the certifications that other personal trainers are going in for.

• Scrutinize the course details of the certifying organizations that you are considering.

• You could also consult personal trainers who are your role-models.

Given below are some of the major certifying organizations and some of the courses that they offer:

American Council on Exercise (ACE):

- Group Fitness Instructor Certification

- Lifestyle & Weight Management Consultant Certification

- Clinical Exercise Specialist Certification

- Peer Fitness Trainer Certification Program

AFAA (Aerobics and Fitness Association of America):

- AFFA Personal Trainer/Fitness Counselor Certification

American College of Sports Medicine (ACSM):

- Health & Fitness Instructor

- ACSM Exercise Specialist

- ACSM Registered Clinical Exercise Physiologist

National Strength & Conditioning Association (NSCA):

- Certified Strength & Conditioning Specialist (CSCS)

- NSCA-Certified Personal Trainer (**NSCA CPT**)

National Academy of Sports Medicine (NASM):

- Performance Enhancement Specialist

National Federation of Professional Trainers (NFPT):

- Certified Athletic Trainer

Issues to Consider

When deciding on the organization where you study to obtain your credentials, consider these issues:

• **Accreditation:** Check to see if the training and/or certifying organization is accredited, and by whom. It's a good idea to also check into the accreditation agency to determine how they set standards and what sort of reputation they have.

• **Club requirements:** If you are going to contract with a club or spa to provide their personal training services, they may require that you and the trainers on your staff be certified through specific organizations. Find out what they prefer before investing in a program they won't accept.

• **Your goals:** Be sure the certification is something you can use and is in line with the goals and aspirations you have for yourself and your company.

• **Your market**: The certification should be appropriate for the market segment you want to serve.

• **Your educational needs**: Some certifying organizations offer only testing programs that determine skills and competency; others offer training programs that lead to certification. Your own needs will determine which you choose.

No matter which certification you choose, make sure that you study to pass the exam. Certification exams are built on rigorous and standardized criteria. That's the only way you can prove that you have what it takes to be a trainer. And if you think that by getting certified you have reached that first milestone, remember that some organizations will require you to be certified in CPR and Advanced First Aid as well. For this, contact your local fire department for a schedule of CPR and First Aid classes. When you complete a class, you will be issued a card to show that you are certified.

Chapter 4

Stand Apart From the Crowd

Who Will You Train?

With more and more people looking to hire personal trainers to stay fit, the profile of your customers has become extremely diverse. And most likely, there are a dozen personal trainer studios in your area to cater to their needs. In this scenario, the big challenge for you is to stand apart from the crowd, to draw customers. For that, you need to start doing things differently.

To begin with decide the client profile that you want to target to. Do you want to work with healthy adults, kids / teens, senior citizens, pregnant women? Once you know the target audience profile, revisit the issue of certification. Are you aware of any specific training methods for your target audience? If not, get certified to train them.

Find Your Niche

Fitness industry is extremely client-centric. Obviously, customer satisfaction is going to be the core of your business. The simple strategy behind a successful personal training business is to,

- Recruit clients
- Service clients for results and value
- Retain clients

So, begin by examining the concept of niche marketing. The question that you should ask here is – what is a niche?

Niche is the specialty or forte that you choose for your business in order to fill an unmet customer need. Typically, you would also be making an effort to match your unique skills to the market needs. For example, you are comfortable using portable equipment in clients' homes. However, you live in a far away suburb, and the sparsely populated market may not be able to support your business. In such a situation, you might decide to explore markets for corporate facilities or offering personal training services in health clubs.

Niches are important because they fulfill specific customer needs that have been ignored, overlooked, or neglected by others. When you choose a niche, you are eliminating competition and ensuring success for your business. And in doing so you are giving a competitive advantage for your business – lack of money, connections, experience notwithstanding.

So, how do you go about creating a niche for your personal training business? Well, now that you know that niche marketing is the exact opposite of mass marketing, scrutinize the other personal training facilities in your area. Find answers to critical questions such as:

1. What is their typical customer profile?

2. Is their any specific customer profile whose needs are left unfulfilled? For example, senior citizens or those with specialized needs?

3. Do you have the certification to cater to this niche group?

4. What services can you offer to this group that other studios don't offer?

Perhaps the senior citizens would like to engage a personal trainer who could train them at their homes? Remember, specialized skills are paid the most. Customers are willing to pay for specialized services that address their specific needs. So if you focus your skills on a niche segment of the industry rest assured that you are sowing the seed of success.

Here's a quick 3-step niche marketing plan for you:

1. Define who you will serve

2. Market to that clientele

3. Provide them with continuing, outstanding service.

The customer profile you choose will impact many aspects of your business like the certification you have chosen, the equipment you buy the work hours that you will keep...

Chapter 5

Price It Right

How Much Will You Charge?

Setting fees and creating billing procedures are critical steps when starting your own business. In a fragmented industry, personal trainers charge anything from $40 to $150 a session. The fee you will set depends on your specialty, skills, experience and the clientele that you aim to build. What you must remember here is that you are offering your customer a service not a product. When buying a car or a television, you know exactly what you are buying and what you can expect from the product. When buying the services of a personal trainer, clients pay for the efficacy of your service and how well you are able to meet their expectations.

Here is a quick checklist that you might want to consider before setting your price:

1. Will you be going to clients' homes for training, or are you considering signing contract with health clubs, or are you looking to train corporate clients?

2. What are your competitors charging in your target market?

3. What are their credentials?

4. What services do they offer?

5. What is the rate variance in this niche segment?

6. Are you open to offering group discounts?

Note: You cannot match your rates to health clubs which have higher volumes and therefore lower rates. It is best to look at independent trainer like yourself.

When you have completed your market research,

1. Do some quick calculations to see how much it will cost you to offer a particular service, for example, your travel cost to the client's home, expenditure on equipment, or if you plan to spend on updating your knowledge at regular intervals. This is your operating cost.

2. Next, determine the annual income you want.

3. Your overheads and your desired income together will give you your annual net income.

4. Now determine how many hours you can work per week. Remember that a club trainer is able

to put in more work hours every week than an independent trainer who spends a sizeable number of hours traveling.

5. Based on this, calculate the total number of hours you will be training per year.

6. Divide your annual net income with the number of hours to figure out the hourly fee you will need to charge. Again, do a quick sanity check to see how this figure compares with the "current rate" for trainers in our market area. And remember, while established trainers can charge slightly higher fees, as a new trainer. You would be better off with offering group packages or even slightly below average rates initially.

Chapter 6

Spread the Word

So you have got your certification, trained your sight on a niche segment, even set your fees after a rigorous market research, but how do you get customers to walk through the door? Advertising your services is the key here. No, we are not suggesting the glitzy million dollar ad campaigns that bring in customers for big businesses. There are in fact many tried and tested ways of silently promoting your business, all the while keeping in mind that what you are essentially doing is to help your client improve their fitness levels.

Most trainers will tell you that word of mouth is the most effective – and cheapest – way of raising awareness. But it may not be sufficient always. So, before you go public with your business think of a name that aptly describes the services that you offer or your vision. Next design a logo that goes well with that name, and print your business cards. Remember, to hand out business cards to all customers – many will have friends who are interested.

Armed with this, you are ready to spread the good word.

1. **Attract Media Attention**: Prepare a press release. If you are not confident of doing a good job of it, hire a professional.

Write a press-release

So you have something to tell the public about your new-found venture, and you want to persuade the media to print it. Here are four simple rules to remember when writing your press release.

a. Headline

With literally hundreds of press releases sitting on the editor's desk, how are you going to make yours stand out? The key lies in writing an attention-grabbing headline. Write it like you were writing a billboard on the highway – few words, dynamic idea that holds attention.

b. Opening Paragraph

Once you have the editor's eyeballs, quickly summarize your story in the opening paragraph. Ensure that it covers all the elements of a good story – the who, what, when, where, why, and how, without going into too much detail.

c. Body Text

Now that he is reading, start adding details. Write the most important information and quotes first. This is the inverted pyramid strategy. This strategy helps you to communicate the most important facts to the end-reader, even if the editor decides to cut your press release for reasons such as space constraints.

d. **The Closing Paragraph**

Finally, repeat your contact information along with the name of your business for better recall.

2. **Conduct Seminars**: Seminars are a good way to boost your image as an expert. And when you organize a free seminar, you will find that people are more than willing to attend programs where they learn new information.

a. Be sure to choose a subject that you are expert in.

b. Then think of interesting ways to supplement your talk, for example with demonstration or information about supplementing an exercise routine with a diet plan.

c. Choose a venue that's easily accessible for your potential clients.

Hone Your Public-speaking Skills

Effective speaking is to project a more confident image, increase your visibility and expand your personal power and presence.

a. Positive Body Language: Drooping shoulders, crossed arms, darting glances, averted eyes are all signs of a poor self-image. Practice positive body signs such as looking your audience in the eye.

b. Preparation is the key to overcoming nervousness. Know your subject well. Decide what information you want to share with your audience.

c. Be certain that your communication is logical and sequential. Create phrases that help transition and connect your ideas. Lead your audience from one idea to the next.

d. Involve your audience in the communication process. Effective listening is part of effective communicating. Ask a question, listen and process their answer.

e. Control the flow of the communication. If someone has overtaken your "turn" to communicate your information, insert yourself back into the control position.

f. Create a powerful closing to your part in the conversation or presentation. Wrap it up and ensure that other know that you have finished speaking and have been listening to you.

g. Ask follow up questions to ensure clarity. Make conclusion statements. Monitor their behavioral reaction to your communication. Ask them in your communication with them was valuable

h. Practice makes perfect. Seize opportunities to make a powerful impression and deliver valuable content.

3. **Get Referrals:** Word of mouth publicity is the best way of advertisement. Satisfied customers are mobile advertisements for your business. They not only build credibility for you, they are also most likely to convert a potential (perhaps a good friend of theirs) into client for you.

4. **Get Published**: Consider writing fitness articles for local newspapers. Your byline is bound to project you as an expert to your readers, potential customers among them.

5. **Offer Free Sessions**: For example, if you are planning to train kids or teens, offer free sessions at schools.

6. **Print flayers, brochures, newsletters** to let others know about your services.

Flayers are an inexpensive and easy way to advertise your business or promotion to prospective clients.

Brochures are appropriate to communicate your company history; announce new programs, products, and services; generate interest in upcoming training and seminars etc.

Newsletters are great for communicating with a group's members e.g., people who have filled out your initial enquiry forms but not enrolled yet. Through newsletters, you can reach out to them and announce new courses, new services etc.

7. **You, yourself:** And last but not the least, what better advertisement than you yourself? Wear a tee printed with your trade name and logo to the local store, on the beach, at the ground.

Chapter 7

Get Equipped

Before you invest in fitness equipment for your new business, it would be wise to remember that at this point of time your cash flow is limited. You cannot afford to lock your resources in equipment that you may never use. What use would be a state-of-the-art treadmill if you are planning to train customers at their location? If you don't intend lugging it over to your customer's home or office thrice a week, then you are saddled with a monster that you may never use after all!

There are many other factors that will influence the kind of equipment you should buy – your budget, available space, the specific needs of our niche market. List your needs diligently and then carefully select the fitness equipment that most suits your requirements, and then look around for equipment that is simple to use, versatile, easy to store and reasonably priced.

Treadmills

Treadmills are easy to use and versatile. Look for models that can be folded.

Average price range: $599 - $2000

Exercise bikes

Cycling is a great cardiovascular workout as it puts less strain on the back, knees and leg joints, improves stamina and promotes lower body conditioning. The upright model most closely mimics outdoor bicycles.

Average Price Range: $599 and above.

Elliptical trainers

Ellipticals or cross trainers are low impact and burn more calories in less time. Many models fold up for easy storage.

Average Price Range: $599 and above

Stair Stepper

Stair steppers offer a good cardiovascular workout in a small space with low join impact.

Average price range: $80 - $150

Rowing machines

A seated aerobic exercise, rowing machines remove all the body weight from the ankles, knees and hips. Many of the models can be folded to half their size, saving on space.

Average price range: $229 - $2500

Dumbbells

Look for a mix of small weights, 10 lb (4.5 kg) and 20 lb (9 kg) hand-held dumbbells and a bar with larger, exchangeable weights, either metal or plastic weights.

Average price range: under $50

Exercise ball

Exercise ball is an excellent way to tighten and tone the entire body.

Whichever equipment you decide to buy, here are some pointers for you:

1. Which of these machines will best help you accomplish your business goals?

2. Do you have the space to accommodate the equipment you are buying?

3. If you are buying from a catalog or television ad, are you thoroughly familiar with the product you are going to spend on?

4. Are you buying a specific model because of its utility and versatility, or because it's trendy?

5. Is the model that you selected easily adjustable to suit needs of different customers?

6. And finally, have you checked the warranty? This piece of paper is invaluable if the equipment you buy turns out to be defective

Chapter 8

Record Keeping

And now, time for number crunching! Account keeping and financials are an important part of any business, especially if you hope to grow your business. Agreed that you decided to become a personal trainer because you enjoy training, but maintaining files and records is integral to any business.

Well maintained and accurate records will help you easily handle the business cash flow and maximize profitability. So no matter how big or small you area the moment, record keeping is essential, especially if you remember that come April and the tax man will be knocking at your door.

So, keep records of payments and expenses. If you are unsure of developing accounting methods, consider hiring a bookkeeper. It is far less expensive to pay a bookkeeper, than accountants, and they can still implement a good record keeping system, handle financial transactions, and produce financial statements for you. Remember that your ledgers are the tools you will need to check the financial health of your business. Both when you are paying taxes and when you are looking for a loan.

If cash flow planning and balance sheets make your head spin, here's some quick help:

1. Open an account for your business transactions.

2. Use checks to make and receive payments.

3. Use invoices for maintaining your sales records.

Chapter 9

When a Client Walks In

So you have publicized your business, documented your policies, even planned good record keeping policies. And now you are all set for that first client to walk through the door.

What do you do now? Quite simply, motivate them to join your one-on-one training program. Remember after all the pre planning that has gone into your business, this is the time for making a sale! Follow the three-step process:

1. **Establish rapport**

   • Use ice-breaking questions

   •Use phrases such as "Tell me more" or "I understand" to encourage the client to share his thoughts and advance your sales process

   • Listen to find out what they need from you

   • Take notes

2. To verify **your understanding of the client's** health goals, repeat what the client has told you.

3. **Explain the programs** that you can offer to answer their specific needs. Also explain the billing

policies, cancellation procedures etc. at this point of time.

The 1st Training Session

So you have converted the prospect into a sale. And now is the time to plan your first session.

You will invest this session in a routine but essential activity–assessing the fitness levels of your client. You will typically start them off on the weighing scales. Next, the girth measurements, followed by measuring blood pressure and body composition. Once you have made your notes, you will start with the fitness assessment.

1. Cardio-vascular endurance

2. Flexibility

3. Muscular strength

Based on these findings, you will now design the training strategy for your client.

1. Is it going to be a strength training routine or an aerobic workout?

2. What equipment will you use?

3. What exercises will you choose?

4. What will be the order of exercises?

5. What will be their intensity and frequency?

6. What will be the volume of the workout?

The answers to these questions will be the start of a healthy relationship between your client and you from the second session onward.

Chapter 10

A Complete Experience

A great way to expand your growing business is to add-on related services or products that satisfy a client-need outside the scope of your current business capabilities. The most logical add-ons for a fitness business are:

a. Massage services

b. Nutrition consultation

Massage Services

You will need certification before you can offer massage therapy to rejuvenate your client's muscles. Find out about the specialized training and schooling requirements in order to legally adding this lucrative service to your fitness business.

Nutrition Supplements

Most likely, many of your clients will have weight-loss as their health goal. If you are a smart entrepreneur, you will identify an opportunity here and add nutrition supplements to your menu. In addition to selling them protein powders and vitamin supplements, you could also consider providing them with nutritional counseling. Just find out your state's legal requirements to practice dietetics, and you are on.

Other add-on ideas for your fitness business could be selling fitness equipment or fitness apparel. Whatever mode you choose to supplement your income, just make sure that it is in line with the basic service that you offer.

Chapter 11

Get, Set, Go!

That brings us to that crucial stage, where you are ready to take the leap. Having gone through every pains taking detail of how to start and sustain your personal trainer business, you are now ready to turn your dream into reality.

But just before you close this book, and launch that high-profile, high-growth, and highly profitable venture, some quick tips:

1. Hone your communication and business skills

2. Update yourself on new technologies and knowledge regularly at least twice a year by attending courses and seminars run by industry bodies. If possible, undergo training in a range of fitness areas to keep your options open. As your business grows, you might want to train a diverse range of customer profiles

3. No matter what, always ensure dependable service for your clients

4. Listen to them with empathy and understanding. Remember, communication is a two-way process; you get to talk, but so do your clients. And when you listen to them, you are able to get feedback about their needs, satisfaction levels, and where your business is headed.

5. Your own fitness levels are crucial to inspire potential customers. When they see a fit, healthy and energetic you, they are willing to see you as a role-model and train with you.

Chapter 12

Forms and Policies

Now is the time for some paperwork. When you are doing business, documentation is crucial to your survival. From simple data sheets to collect information about a potential customer to accident report forms, you should have your paperwork in order. In an injury-prone occupation such as personal training, this is the only way to stay out of litigations.

Given below is a list of forms and policies that will help you create a small consultation packet for initial meetings with the client:

- Initial consultation sheet

- Medical history form

- Exercise history form

- Packages and pricing sheet

- Cancellation Policy

- Refund Policy

- Waiver of liability

Here are some basic forms that you could use. You can also download those forms and print or edit them by going to my web site:

www.personaltrainerjob.com/forms

Informed consent and waiver

I,_____, do hereby consent to participate in a personal training program that will include weight training and or cardiovascular exercise. I have been informed and understand that physical exercise has been associated with certain risks, including but not limited to musculoskeletal injury, spinal injuries, abnormal blood pressure responses, and, in rare instances, heart attack or death. Every effort will be made to minimize these risks.

Any information that is obtained regarding my fitness level and my progress will be treated as privileged and confidential and will not be released or revealed to any person other than my physician or the program's Supervisor (for record keeping purposes) without my expressed written consent.

I have read and understand the foregoing consent to participation in said program. I am aware that I may discontinue participation in the program at any time that I see fit to do so. If at any time I have questions concerning the content, policies, or procedures regarding the personal training program (One-On-One Fitness) I will discuss these questions with my trainer or the program Supervisor immediately.

In addition, I agree to the following:

a) assume all risk of injury and all risk of damage to or loss of property arising out of my participation in this program;

b) release, discharge, and waive any and all responsibility of the _____ from and against any liability of injury, including death, and for damage to or loss of property which may be suffered by the undersigned arising out of, or in any way connected with the participation in this program; and

c) indemnify and hold harmless University, its officers, agents and employees from and against all liability, claims, demands, actions, loss, and damage arising out of my participation in said personal training program.

Consenting Signature:

Participant:

Date:

Witness:

Date:

Personal Health History

Name:

Address:

City: State: Zip:

Telephone (Day):   (Evening):

Gender: Age: Date of Birth:

CARDIOVASULAR RISK

Please check any that apply and state the age of onset for the persons named below:

You Mother Father Grandparent

High Blood Pressure:

High Cholesterol:

Diabetes:

Heart Disease:

Bypass Surgery:

Stroke:

Do you presently smoke cigarettes?
If yes, how many per day?

Have you ever quit smoking?
If yes, how long ago did you quit?

Height

Current Weight

PERSONAL HISTORY

Date of last physical examination

Stress Test

Resting EKG

Date of last blood cholesterol test

Total Serum Cholesterol

HDL

Date of last blood pressure test
Blood Pressure

Has you doctor ever restricted your physical activity?
If yes, please explain

Do you have any allergies?
If yes, please list

Do you ever experience chest pains or tightness?

Do you ever experience unusual shortness of breath during mild physical activity?

Are you presently taking any medication?
If yes, please list type and purpose

Do you ever experience dizziness during vigorous physical activity?

Have you ever passed out during vigorous physical activity?

Do you have any (other) medical conditions which limit your ability to exercise?
If yes, please explain

If you are female, are you currently pregnant?

INJURIES

Please check any of the following injuries you have had and specify which bone, muscle, joint, etc., and the year the injury occurred:

Broken bones

Muscle strain/sprain

Ligament, tendon, or cartilage injury

Joint injury or chronic pain

Back injury or chronic pain

Other

Are you currently being treated for any of the above injuries?
If yes, please specify the type of treatment

LIFESTYLE

Are you:

• Generally sedentary

• Weekend or vacation exerciser

• Physically active once or twice a week

•Physically active more often

Do you currently have a regular exercise program?
If yes, please describe:

TRAINING INTEREST AND GOALS

Please check any activities in which you are interested in participating:

- Weight training

- Aerobics

- Rowing

- Stairmaster

- Running

- Stationary bike

- Swimming

- Triathlons

- Walking

- Other (Specify)

How much time do you want to spend working out?

Do you have any exercise equipment at home?

Do you feel that there are any specific exercises that would not interest you or might cause you pain or discomfort?

What goals do you have concerning your training and health?

Signature:

Date:

PAR – Q (Physical Activity Readiness – Questionnaire)

If you are a man over the age of 45 or a woman over the age of 55 you are required to complete a "Medical Authorization Form" BEFORE training.

I have read, understood and completed this questionnaire. Any questions I had were answered to my full satisfaction.

NAME:

DATE:

SIGNATURE:

WITNESS:
YES / NO

1. Has your doctor ever said that you have a heart condition and that you should only do physical activity recommended by a doctor?

2. Do you feel pain in your chest when you do physical activity?

3. In the past month, have you had chest pain when you were not doing physical activity?

4. Do you lose your balance because of izziness or do you ever lose consciousness?

5. Do you have a bone or joint problem that could be made worse by a change in your physical activity?

6. Is your doctor currently prescribing drugs (for example, water pills) your blood pressure or heart condition?

7. Do you know of any other reason why you should not do physical activity?

NOTE:

1. Tell your doctor about the PAR-Q and which questions you answered YES. Talk with your doctor about the kinds of activities you wish to participate in and follow his/he advice.

2. If you are or may be pregnant – talk with your doctor before you start becoming more active.

Client Exercise History Questionnaire

Name:

DOB:

Date:

Address:

Home Number:

Work Number:

Cell Number:

Fax Number:

E-mail address:

Occupation:

How many hours of week do you work?

Contact in case of emergency:

Married/single:

Current Weight:

How long at this weight?

Height:

Have you ever had a personal trainer before and where?

What did you like most about working with them?

What did you like least about working with them?

Describe what you would like to accomplish through your fitness program with me:

Aside from technical knowledge and personal attention, what type of motivation do you require and expect from a trainer?

What can we do together to make your exercise program more enjoyable? Do you own any type of exercise equipment? (Please list):

What are your current leisure activities?

Would you be interested in learning more about fitness, nutrition and lifestyle weight management through reading, watching a video, or listening to an audio cassette?

Please rate your exercise level on a scale of 1 – 5 (5 indicating very strenuous) for each age range through your present age range:
▫13-20 ▫21-30 ▫ 31-40 ▫41-50 ▫50±

Were you (or are you)a high school or college athlete? If yes, please specify:

Do you have negative feelings toward, or have you ever had any bad experience with a physical activity program? If yes, please explain:

Rate yourself on scale of 1 to 5 (1 indicating the lowest value). Check the appropriate box number that best applies:

Characterize your present athletic ability.
▫01 ▫02 ▫03 ▫04 ▫05

When you exercise, how important is competition?
▫01 ▫02 ▫03 ▫04 ▫05

Characterize your present cardiovascular capacity.
▫01 ▫02 ▫03 ▫04 ▫05

Characterize your present muscular capacity.
▫01 ▫02 ▫03 ▫04 ▫05

Characterize your present flexibility capacity.
▫01 ▫02 ▫03 ▫04 ▫05

Do you start exercise programs but then find yourself unable to stick with them? No Yes, please describe barriers:

How much time are you willing to devote to an exercise program?

Are you currently involved in regular endurance (cardiovascular) exercise?
▫No   ▫Yes, specify type(s) of exercise:

Rate your perception of the exertion of your exercise program. (Please check appropriate box):

▫Light ▫Fairly light ▫Somewhat hard ▫Hard

How long have you been exercising regularly?

What other exercise, sports or recreational activities have you participated in?

In the past 6 months?

In the past 5 years?

What types of exercise interests you? (Please check all applicable.)

▫Walking (treadmill/outdoors)

- Running (treadmill/outdoors)

- Hiking

- Swimming

- Tennis

- Golf

- Cycling

- Stationary biking
- Spin classer owing

- Strength training

- Softball/baseball

- Martial arts

- Tai Chi

- Yoga

- Stretching

- Pilates

- Dance

Use the following scale to rate each goal as far as an exercise program:

▫Not at all Important ▫Somewhat Important ▫Extremely Important
1   2   3   4   5   6   7   8   9   10

Improve cardiovascular fitness:

Body-fat weight loss

Reshape or tone my body

Build more muscle:

Improve flexibility

Increase strength

Increase energy level:

Improve performance for a specific sport:

Improve mood and ability to cope with stress:

Feel better/improved health:

Enjoyment:

Anything else I should know about you?

Signature:

Date:

Health Questionnaire

Name:

Date:

1. Have you ever had heart trouble or coronary disease? If so please explain:

2. Do you have a family history of heart problems or coronary disease? If yes please explain:

3. Do you have a history of high blood pressure (above 140/90)?

4. Do you have diabetes?

Please provide name and phone number of your doctor:

5. Do you think you are overweight?

6. Has your doctor ever said you have high cholesterol?

7. Please list any prescribed medications you are taking:

8. Please list any drug allergies:

9. Please list any over the counter medication or dietary supplements you are taking:

10. Please list any illness, hospitalization, or surgical procedure within the past 3 years:

11. Please list date of last physical examination and results.

12 .Are you currently under a care of a physician?

If so, please describe and provide name and phone number of your doctor:

13. Do you have trouble sleeping?

How many hours of sleep per night?

14. Do you wear eyeglasses or contacts?

15. How many cups of coffee _____ soda _____ water do you drink a day

17. Have you ever participated in a diet and/or nutrition program?

Did you achieve your goal(s)?

Was it permanent?

18. What would you like to change about your health or the way you look?

19. Have you ever been treated for, diagnosed as having, or currently suffering from any of the following: (Explain below for each "Yes")
Yes
No

Skin tumors, skin cancer or melanoma?
Yes
No

Cancer?
Yes
No

Any infectious progressive illness, such as Hepatitis B, Acquired Immune Deficiency Syndrome or other conditions?
Yes
No

Are you currently under the care of a physical therapist?
Yes
No

Any circulatory disorder
Yes
No

Neuromuscular /neurological disorders such as seizures?
Yes
No
Suffered from fainting, convulsions, recurrent headaches, and dizziness?
Yes
No

Stroke?
Yes
No

Nervous or mental disorder?
Yes
No

Active rheumatoid arthritis?
Yes
No

Osteoporosis?
Yes
No

Anti-coagulant medication?
Yes
No

Are you taking anti-depressive medication?
Yes
No

Are you under hormonal treatment?
Yes
No

Liposuction or cosmetic surgery within the last six months?
Yes
No

Allergies?
Yes
No

Digestive problems?
Yes
No

Are you taking laxatives or diuretics?
Yes
No

Do you smoke? How many cigarettes a day?
Yes
No

Are you pregnant?

Yes
No

Signature:

Date:

Waiver & Release Form

Because physical exercise can be strenuous and subject to risk of serious injury, we urge you to obtain a physical examination from a doctor before using any exercise equipment or participating in any exercise activity.

ou agree that by participating in physical exercise or training activities, you do so entirely at your own risk. Any recommendation for changes in diet including the use of food supplements, eight reduction and/or body building enhancement products are entirely your responsibility and you should consult a physician prior to undergoing any dietary or food supplement changes.

ou agree that you are voluntarily participating in these activities and use of these facilities and premises and assume all risks of injury, illness, or death. We are also not responsible for any loss of your personal property.

You acknowledge that you have carefully read this "waiver and release" and fully understand that it is a release of liability. You expressly agree to release and discharge the trainer or instructor from any and all claims or causes of action and you agree to voluntarily give up or waive any right that you may otherwise have to bring a legal action against the trainer or instructor for personal injury or property damage.

To the extent that statute or case law does not prohibit releases for negligence, this release is also for negligence.

If any portion of this release from liability shall be deemed by a Court of competent jurisdiction to be invalid, then the remainder of this release from liability shall remain in full force and effect and the offending provision or provisions severed here from.

By signing this release, I acknowledge that I understand its content and that this release cannot be modified orally.

Signature:_____

Date:_____

And finally here are some tips for you to determine the billing and cancellation policies:

1. It works best if you keep a pre-pay policy for all billing.

2. Work on a scheduled appointment basis. Ask the clients to give you a minimum of 24-hour notice to cancel an appointment. This will help you schedule another customer.

3. Alternately, if you have to cancel an appointment for some reason, ensure that you reschedule the appointment at a later time according to the client's convenience.

Where To Buy This Book

You can buy this book on Amazon. Just go to amazon.com (or your local Amazon site if available) and search for "How To Become A Certified Personal Trainer by Joe Dynasty" or just "Joe Dynasty".

You can also order it at any bookstore if they don't have it in stock. Just give them the IBSN below:

ISBN 978-0-9866004-3-2

Latest Books by Psylon Press

Forever Laid Formula
Best Ways To Get Women To Sleep With You
By Taylor Timms
ISBN 978-0-9866004-2-5

Best Gift Ideas For Women
By Taylor Timms
ISBN 978-0-9866004-4-9

100% Blonde Jokes
The Best Dumb, Funny, Clean, Short and
Long Blonde Jokes Book
By R. Cristi
ISBN 978-0-9866004-1-8

www.ingramcontent.com/pod-product-compliance
Lightning Source LLC
Chambersburg PA
CBHW070856280326
41934CB00008B/1467

9 780986 600432